Frequently Asked Questions
PROSTHODONTICS

Frequently Asked Questions
PROSTHODONTICS

*A free companion to
Essential Quick Review: Prosthodontics*

Editor-in-Chief
Priya Verma Gupta MDS FPFA
Professor
Department of Paedodontics and Preventive Dentistry
Divya Jyoti College of Dental Sciences and Research
Ghaziabad, Uttar Pradesh, India

Co-Author
Suraj R Suvarna MDS
Professor
Department of Prosthodontics
Shree Bankey Bihari Dental College and Research Centre
Masuri, Uttar Pradesh, India

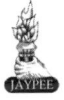

The Health Sciences Publisher
New Delhi | London | Philadelphia | Panama

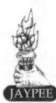

Jaypee Brothers Medical Publishers (P) Ltd

Headquarters
Jaypee Brothers Medical Publishers (P) Ltd
4838/24, Ansari Road, Daryaganj
New Delhi 110 002, India
Phone: +91-11-43574357
Fax: +91-11-43574314
Email: jaypee@jaypeebrothers.com

Overseas Offices

J.P. Medical Ltd
83 Victoria Street, London
SW1H 0HW (UK)
Phone: +44 20 3170 8910
Fax: +44 (0)20 3008 6180
Email: info@jpmedpub.com

Jaypee-Highlights Medical Publishers Inc.
City of Knowledge, Bld. 235, Clayton
Panama City, Panama
Phone: +1 507-301-0496
Fax: +1 507-301-0499
Email: cservice@jphmedical.com

Jaypee Medical Inc.
325 Chestnut Street
Suite 412, Philadelphia,
PA 19106, USA
Phone: +1 267-519-9789
Email: support@jpmedus.com

Jaypee Brothers Medical Publishers (P) Ltd
17/1-B Babar Road, Block-B, Shaymali
Mohammadpur, Dhaka-1207
Bangladesh
Mobile: +08801912003485
Email: jaypeedhaka@gmail.com

Jaypee Brothers Medical Publishers (P) Ltd
Bhotahity, Kathmandu, Nepal
Phone: +977-9741283608
Email: kathmandu@jaypeebrothers.com

Website: www.jaypeebrothers.com
Website: www.jaypeedigital.com

© 2017, Jaypee Brothers Medical Publishers

The views and opinions expressed in this book are solely those of the original contributor(s)/author(s) and do not necessarily represent those of editor(s) of the book.

All rights reserved. No part of this publication may be reproduced, stored or transmitted in any form or by any means, electronic, mechanical, photocopying, recording or otherwise, without the prior permission in writing of the publishers.

All brand names and product names used in this book are trade names, service marks, trademarks or registered trademarks of their respective owners. The publisher is not associated with any product or vendor mentioned in this book.

Medical knowledge and practice change constantly. This book is designed to provide accurate, authoritative information about the subject matter in question. However, readers are advised to check the most current information available on procedures included and check information from the manufacturer of each product to be administered, to verify the recommended dose, formula, method and duration of administration, adverse effects and contraindications. It is the responsibility of the practitioner to take all appropriate safety precautions. Neither the publisher nor the author(s)/editor(s) assume any liability for any injury and/or damage to persons or property arising from or related to use of material in this book.

This book is sold on the understanding that the publisher is not engaged in providing professional medical services. If such advice or services are required, the services of a competent medical professional should be sought.

Every effort has been made where necessary to contact holders of copyright to obtain permission to reproduce copyright material. If any have been inadvertently overlooked, the publisher will be pleased to make the necessary arrangements at the first opportunity.

Inquiries for bulk sales may be solicited at: jaypee@jaypeebrothers.com

Frequently Asked Questions: Prosthodontics

First Edition: **2017**

ISBN: 978-93-86107-80-0

Printed at Rajkamal Electric Press, Plot No. 2, Phase-IV, Kundli, Haryana.

Editorial Board

Priya Verma Gupta MDS FPFA
Professor
Department of Paedodontics and Preventive Dentistry
Divya Jyoti College of Dental Sciences and Research
Modi Nagar, Niwari Road, Ghaziabad
Uttar Pradesh, India

Gunjan Gupta MDS
Assistant Professor
Department of Periodontics
Shree Bankey Bihari Dental College and Research Centre
Hapur Road, Ghaziabad
Uttar Pradesh, India

Nishant Gupta MDS
Assistant Professor
Department of Orthodontics and Dentofacial Orthopedics
Shree Bankey Bihari Dental College and Research Centre
Hapur Road, Ghaziabad
Uttar Pradesh, India

Rishab Malhotra MDS
Assistant Professor
Department of Paedodontics and Preventive Dentistry
Jaipur Dental College
Jaipur, Rajasthan, India

Preface

I am very pleased to introduce you to the first edition of Essential Quick Review; A series for final year undergraduate students.

The series will be available in eight subjects, i.e., Periodontics, Operative Dentistry and Endodontics, Paedodontics, Prosthodontics, Oral Surgery, Oral Medicine and Radiology, Orthodontics and Public Health Dentistry covering essential parts of each subject. This book will not only help the student to attain the knowledge, but will also give an idea how to attempt a question during the examination, covering entire syllabus in a limited period of time.

It is a supplementary booklet for each subject that contains three sections, i.e., definitions, classifications and viva-voce covering the entire syllabus enabling the student to undergo a quick revision. The language used is very simple for better understanding.

The study material provided in this book is an attempt to provide an additional help to students for easy retention and reproduction of subject in the examination. This book is in no way a replacement to standard text book.

I thank all my subject matter experts for their valued suggestions and contributions. A very special word of thanks to my family for being the source of constant encouragement.

I profusely thank Shri Jitendar P Vij (CEO), Mr Ankit Vij (Group President), and production team of M/S Jaypee Brothers Medical Publishers (P) Ltd, New Delhi for their enthusiasm and constant efforts in bringing out this book.

Priya Verma Gupta

Contents

1. Definitions 1-28
2. Classifications 29-40
3. Viva-Voce 41-104

PROSTHODONTICS

Definitions

Complete Denture Prosthodontics

The replacement of the natural teeth in the arch and their associated parts by artificial substitutes.

Aesthetics

It is a pleasure feeling obtained due to visual perception of an object. The complete denture should restore the lost facial contours, vertical dimension, etc. Artefacts like stains can be incorporated in order to improve the aesthetics

Mastication

A complete denture should have proper balanced occlusion in order to enhance the stability of the denture

Phonetics

That portion of the denture surface which has its contour determined by the impression. One of the most important functions of a denture is to restore the speech of the impression surface (Intaglio surface)

Polished Surface (Cameo Surface)

That portion of a surface of a denture which extends in an occlusal direction from the border of the denture and includes the palatal surfaces. It is the part of the denture base which is usually polished. It includes the buccal and lingual surfaces of the teeth

Occlusal Surface

That portion of the surface of a denture or dentition which makes contact or near contact with the corresponding surface of the opposing denture or dentition

Labial Flange

The portion of the flange of the denture which occupies the labial vestibule of the mouth

Buccal Flange

The portion of a flange of a denture which occupies the buccal vestibule of the mouth

Lingual Flange

The portion of the flange of a mandibular denture which occupies the space adjacent to the tongue

Denture Border

The margin of the denture base at the junction of the polished surface and the impression surface

Anatomic Teeth

Teeth which have prominent pointed or rounded cusps on the masticating surfaces. These are designed to occlude with the teeth of the opposing denture or natural dentition

Non-anatomical Teeth

Artificial teeth with occlusal surfaces which are not anatomically formed. These are designed to improve the function of mastication

Cuspless Teeth

Teeth that are designed without cuspal prominences on the occlusal surfaces

Tori

Tori are abnormal bony prominences found in the middle of the palatal vault and on the lingual side of the mandible in the premolar region

Diagnostic Impression

The negative replica of the oral tissues used to prepare a diagnostic cast

Mouth Rehabilitation

A Restoration of the form and function of the masticatory apparatus to as nearly normal as possible

Vestibuloplasty

It is a surgical procedure to increase the vestibular depth

Special Tray

A custom made device prepared for a particular patient which is used to carry, confine and control an impression material while making an impression

Border Moulding or Peripheral Tracing

The shaping of an impression material by manipulation or action of the tissues adjacent to the borders of the impression

Posterior Palatal Seal

The soft tissues along the junction of the hard and soft palates on which pressure within the physiological limits of the tissues can be applied by a denture to aid in the retention of the denture

Beading and Boxing

Beading is done to preserve the width and height of the sulcus in a cast. Boxing is done to obtain a uniform, smooth and well-shaped base for the cast

Occlusal Rim

Occluding surfaces built on temporary or permanent denture bases for the purpose of making maxillomandibular relation records and arranging teeth

Condylar Guidance

Mandibular guidance generated by the condyle and articular disc traversing the contour of the glenoid fossa

Incisal Guidance (Anterior Determinant)

The influence of the contacting surfaces of the mandibular and maxillary anterior teeth during mandibular movements

Incisal Guide Angle

The angle formed in the horizontal plane by drawing a line in the sagittal plane between the incisal edges of the maxillary and mandibular central incisors when the teeth are in centric occlusion. The angle formed between the long axis of the upper and lower anteriors is called the incisal guide angle

Bennett Movement

The bodily lateral movement or lateral shift of the mandible resulting from the movements of the condyles along the lateral inclines along the mandibular fossae in lateral jaw movements

Jaw Relation

Any relation of the mandible to the maxilla

Orientation Relation

The mandible which is kept at its most posterior portion, it can rotate in the sagittal plane around an imaginary transverse axis passing through or near the condyles

Vertical Relation

The amount of separation between the maxilla and mandible in the frontal plane

Horizontal Relation

Maxillomandibular relationship in which the condyles articulate with the thinnest avascular portion of their respective discs with the complex in the anterosuperior direction against the slopes of articular eminence

Centric Jaw Relation

The most posterior relation of the mandible to the maxilla at the established vertical dimension

Eccentric Jaw Relation

Any jaw relation other than centric jaw relation

Median Jaw Relation

Any jaw relation when the mandible is in the median sagittal plane

Posterior Border Jaw Relation

The most posterior relation of the mandible to the maxilla at any specific vertical relation

Protrusive Jaw Relation

A jaw relation resulting from a protrusion of the mandible

Rest Jaw Relation

The habitual postural jaw relation when the patient is resting comfortably in an upright position and the condyles are in a neutral, unrestrained position in the glenoid fossa

Unstrained Jaw Relation

The relation of the mandible to the skull when a state of balanced tonus exists among all the muscles involved. Any jaw relation that is attained without undue or unnatural force and which causes no undue distortion of the tissues of the temporomandibular joint

Jaw Relation Record

A registration of any positional relationship of the mandible in reference to the maxilla. These records may be any of the many vertical, horizontal and orientation relations

Terminal Jaw Relation Record

A record of the relationship of the mandible to the maxilla made at the vertical dimension of occlusion and at the centric relation

Jaw Repositioning

The jaw relation when the mandible is kept in its most posterior position, it can rotate in the sagittal plane around an imaginary transverse axis passing through or near the condyles. The changing of any relative position of the mandible to the maxilla, usually by altering the occlusion of the natural or artificial teeth

Face-bow

A caliper like device which is used to record the relationship of the jaws to the temporomandibular joints and to orient the casts on the articulator to the relationship of the opening axis of the temporomandibular joint

Vertical Jaw Relation

The length of the face as determined by the amount of separation of the jaws

Vertical Dimension at Rest

The length of the face when the mandible is in rest position

Ridge Relation

The positional relationship of the mandibular ridge to the maxillary ridge

Centric Relation

The maxillomandibular relationship in which the condyles articulate with the thinnest avascular portion of their respective discs with the complex in the anterior-superior position against the slopes of the articular eminences. This position is independent of tooth contact. This position is clinically discernible when the mandible is directed superior and anteriorly. It is restricted to a purely rotary movement about the transverse horizontal axis

Central Bearing Point

The contact point of the central bearing device

Pantographic Tracing

A graphic record of mandibular movement in three planes as registered by the styli on the recording tables of a pantograph; tracings of mandibular movement recorded on plates in the horizontal and sagittal planes

Pantographic Tracer

An instrument used to graphically record one or more plane paths of the mandibular movement and to provide information for the programming of the articulator

Eccentric Jaw Relation

Any relationship of the mandible to the maxilla other than the centric relation

Articulator

A mechanical device which represents the temporomandibular joints and the jaw members to which maxillary and mandibular casts may be attached to simulate jaw movements

Incisal Guide Table

That part of the articulator which maintains the incisal guide angle

Squint Test

It is used to check and compare the colour of the teeth with the colour of the face. The dentist should partially close his eyes to reduce light and compare artificial teeth of different shades with the colour of the face. The colour of the teeth that fades first from view is least conspicuous (contrasting) to the colour of the face

Semi-anatomic Teeth

Teeth that are used in cases with mild discrepancies in jaw relation and may have 20° or 10° cuspal angulation. These are also known as modified-cusp or low-cusp teeth. 10° semi-anatomic teeth are commonly known as functional or anatoline teeth

Cuspless Teeth

Teeth with no cuspal angulation, hence are very flexible to set in balanced occlusion. These are also known as 0°, flat and monoplane teeth

Occlusion

Any contact between the incising or masticating surfaces of the maxillary and mandibular teeth

Dental Articulation

The static and dynamic contact relationship between the occlusal surfaces of the teeth during function

Balanced Occlusion

The simultaneous contacting of the maxillary and mandibular teeth on the right and left and in the posterior and anterior occlusal areas in centric and eccentric positions, developed to lessen or limit tipping or rotating of the denture bases in relation to the supporting structures

Inclination of the Condylar Path

It is registered using protrusive registration (i.e. the patient is asked to protrude with the occlusal rims. Inter-occlusal record material is injected between the occlusal rims in this position It is also called as the first factor of occlusion. This is the only factor, which can be recorded from the patient

Plane of Occlusion or Occlusal Plane

An imaginary surface which is related anatomically to the cranium and which theoretically touches the incisal edges of the incisors and the tips of the occluding surfaces of the posterior teeth. It is not a plane in the true sense of the word but represents the mean curvature of the surface

Compensating Curve

The anteroposterior and lateral curvatures in the alignment of the occluding surfaces and incisal edges of artificial teeth which are used to develop balanced occlusion

Curve of Spee

The anatomic curvature of the occlusal alignment of teeth beginning at the tip of the lower canine and following the buccal cusps of the natural premolars and molars, continuing to the anterior border of the ramus as described by Graf Von Spee

Monson's Curve

The curve of occlusion in which each cusp and incisal edge touches or conforms to a segment of a sphere of 8 inches in diameter with its center in the region of the Glabella

Wilson's Curve

A curve of occlusion which is convex upwards

Reverse Curve

A curve of occlusion in which transverse cross-section conforms to a line which is convex upwards

Pleasure Curve

A curve of occlusion in which transverse cross-section conforms to a line which is convex upward except for the last molars

Cuspal Angulation

Cusp angle is defined as the angle made by the average slope of a cusp with the cusp plane measured mesiodistally or buccolingually

Key of Occlusion

It denotes the relationship of the upper and lower teeth during function

Waxing up

The contouring of a pattern in wax generally applied to shaping in wax of the contours of a trial denture

Try-in Verification or Aesthetic Try-in

A preliminary insertion of a removable denture waxup or a partial denture casting or a finished restoration to determine the fit, aesthetics and maxillomandibular relation

Dewaxing

Dewaxing is done to remove the wax in the wax pattern so that a mould space is created for acrylic to fill-in. It is carried out by placing the flask in boiling water (100ºC) for 5 minutes. Before placing the flask into the water bath, the clamp should be loosened. Dewaxing is done to just soften the wax and not melt it

Denture Stomatitis

It is the pathological reaction of the palatal portion of the denture-bearing mucosa. It is commonly known as 'Denture induced stomatitis'

Flabby Ridge

The alveolar ridge may become mobile and extremely resilient due to the replacement of bone by fibrous tissue. Flabby ridges are most commonly seen in the anterior part of maxilla opposing natural mandibular anterior teeth. This is due to the presence of excessive load on the ridge and unstable occlusal conditions. Histopathology reveals marked fibrosis, inflammation and resorption of the underlying bone

Traumatic Ulcers

The small, painful lesions covered with a grey necrotic membrane and surrounded by an inflammatory halo with firm and elevated borders. They are commonly known as 'sore spots'. They usually develop within 1–2 days after placement of new dentures

Denture Irritation Hyperplasia (Epulis Fissuratum)

It is a hyperplastic reaction of the mucosa occurring along the borders of the denture. These lesions result from trauma due to unstable dentures with thin denture flanges

Burning Mouth Syndrome (BMS)

It is characterized by burning sensation in the structures in contact with the dentures without any visible changes in the mucosa. This lesion is different from burning mouth sensation where the mucosa is often inflamed due to mechanical irritation, infection or an allergic reaction. The mucosa is clinically healthy in BMS

Gagging

The gag reflex is a normal, healthy defense mechanism, which functions to prevent foreign bodies from entering the trachea

Residual Ridge Resorption (RRR)

This is the most common and important sequel of wearing complete dentures. It is nothing but alveolar remodeling, which occurs due to change in the functional stimulus of bone tissue

Ridge Resorption

It is a chronic progressive change in the bone structure, which results in severe impairment in the fit and function of the prosthesis

Disuse Atrophy

Atrophy of a muscle due to poor usage is called disuse atrophy

Impression Trays

A device used to carry, confine and control the impression material while making an impression

Impression Material

Any substance, or combination of substances used for making a negative reproduction or impression

Splinting of Abutments

The joining of two or more teeth into a rigid unit by means of fixed restorations

Splint

A prosthesis which maintains a hard and/or soft tissue in a predetermined position

Denture Design

A planned visualization of the form and extent of a dental prosthesis arrived at after a study of all factors involved

Surveyor

An instrument used in the construction of a removable partial denture to locate and delineate the contours and relative positions of abutment teeth and associated structures

Survey Line

A line produced on a cast of a tooth by a surveyor or scriber marking the greatest height of contour in relation to the chosen path of insertion of a planned restoration The survey line marks the height of contour of the tooth

Height of Contour

A line encircling a tooth designating it's greatest circumference at a selected position

Guiding Planes/Guide Planes

Two or more vertically parallel surfaces of abutment teeth so oriented as to direct the path of placement and removal of removable partial dentures

Major Connector

A part of a removable partial denture which connects the components on one side of the arch to the components on the opposite side of the arch

Minor Connector

The connecting link between the major connector or base of a removable partial denture and other units of the prosthesis, such as clasps, indirect retainers and occlusal rests.

Rest

A rigid (stabilizing) extension of a fixed or removable partial denture which contacts a remaining tooth or teeth to dissipate vertical or horizontal forces

Occlusal Rest

A rigid extension of a partial denture which contacts the occlusal surface of the tooth. It transmits stress along the long axis of tooth. A shallow channel like preparation should be prepared on the lingual surface of the abutment for the placement of the minor connector. When multiple incisal rests are placed each one is not individually connected to the major connector. Instead they are interconnected with a metal plate which is connected to the major connector

Direct Retainer

It is that component part of a removable partial denture that is used to retain and prevent dislodgement, consisting of a clasp assembly or precision attachment. A clasp or attachment applied to an abutment tooth for the purpose of holding a removable denture in position

Retention

Retention is that quality inherent in the prosthesis which resists the force of gravity, the adhesiveness of foods and the forces associated with the opening of the jaws

Direct Retention

Retention obtained in a removable partial denture by the use of clasps or attachments which resist removal from the abutment teeth

Indirect Retention

Retention obtained in a removable partial denture through the use of indirect retainers

Extracoronal Direct Retainer

A part of a removable partial denture which acts as a direct retainer and/or stabilizer for the denture by partially encircling or contacting an abutment tooth

Retentive Arm

A flexible segment of a removable partial denture which engages an undercut on an abutment and is designed to retain the denture

Reciprocal Arm

A clasp arm or other extension used on a removable partial denture to oppose the action of some other part or parts of the prosthesis

Rest

A rigid (stabilizing) extension of a removable partial denture which contacts a remaining tooth or teeth to dissipate vertical or horizontal forces

Minor Connector

The connecting link between the major connector or base of a removable partial denture and other units of the prosthesis such as clasps, indirect retainers and occlusal rests

Retention

Retention is that quality inherent in the prosthesis which resists the force of gravity, the adhesiveness of foods, and the forces associated with the opening of the jaws

Path of Insertion

The direction in which a prosthesis is placed upon and removed from the abutment teeth

Stability

The quality of a denture to be firm, steady, or constant, to resist displacement by functional stresses and not to be subjected to change of position when forces are applied

Support

To hold up or serve as a foundation or prop for. It is the resistance to the movement of the denture in a gingival direction (along the path of insertion)

Reciprocation

The means by which one part of a prosthesis is made to counter the effect created by another part

Passivity

The quality or condition of inactivity or rest assumed by the teeth, tissues and denture when a removable partial denture is in place but not under masticatory pressure

Retainer

The fixation device or any form of attachment applied directly to an abutment tooth and used for the fixation of a prosthesis is called as retainer.e.g clasps. In fixed partial dentures, it refers to a crown that is used as a part of the fixed partial denture for retention and support from the abutment tooth

Definitions

Indirect Retainer

A part of a removable partial denture which assists the direct retainers in preventing displacement of distal extension denture bases by functioning through lever action on the opposite side of the fulcrum line

Retentive Fulcrum Line

An imaginary line, connecting the retentive points of clasp arms, around which the denture tends to rotate when subjected to forces, such as the pull of sticky foods

Stabilizing Fulcrum Line

An imaginary line, connecting occlusal rests, around which the denture tends to rotate under masticatory forces It is easy to lift a bar with a single support as it will act like a fulcrum and allow free rotation of the bar

Primary Abutment

A tooth used for the direct support of a fixed or removable dental prosthesis

Denture Base

The part of a denture which rests on the oral mucosa and to which teeth are attached. In others words, that part of a complete or removable partial denture which rests upon the basal seat and to which teeth are attached

Tube Teeth

Artificial teeth with an internal, vertical and cylindrical aperture extending from the center of the base upward into the body of the tooth into which a pin may be placed or cast for the attachment of the tooth to a denture (fixed or removable) base

Forces of Adhesion

The physical attraction of unlike molecules for one another

Forces of Cohesion

The physical attraction of like molecules for one another

Stress Breaker

A device which relieves the abutment teeth of all or part of the occlusal forces

Enameloplasty

The intentional alteration of the occlusal surface of the teeth to change their form

Design Transfer

It is defined as, conveying the outline of the proposed prosthesis from the diagnostic cast to the master cast

Blockout

Elimination of undesirable under cut areas on the cast to be used in the fabrication of the removable partial denture

Relief

The procedure of placing a sheet of wax in strategic areas on the master cast to be duplicated so that a refractory cast can be made

Beading

Scoring a cast with a sharp instrument or bur in any desired area to provide a seal between the finished prosthesis and the soft tissue obtain a metal framework

Investing

The process of covering or enveloping, wholly or in part, an object such as a denture, tooth, wax form, crown, etc. with a suitable investment material before processing, soldering or casting

Overdenture

It is a denture that may be supported by soft tissue, bone, root of a tooth or a modified tooth

Unilateral Removable Partial Dendure

A dental prosthesis restoring lost or missing teeth on one side of the arch only

Temporary Partial Denture

A dental prosthesis to be used for a short interval of time for aesthetics, mastication, occlusal support or convenience or to condition the patient to the acceptance of an artificial substitute for missing natural teeth until more definitive prosthetic therapy can be provided

Transitional Partial Denture

A removable partial denture serving as a temporary prosthesis to which artificial teeth will be added as natural teeth are lost and which will be replaced after post-extraction tissue changes have occurred

Interim Partial Denture

A transitional denture may become an interim denture when all of the natural teeth have been removed from the dental arch

Treatment Partial Denture

A dental prosthesis used for the purpose of treating or conditioning the tissues which are called upon to support and retain a denture base

Relining

It is defined as to resurface the tissue side of a denture base with new base material to make the denture fit more accurately

Rebasing

A process of refitting a denture by the replacement of the denture-base material

Fixed Partial Denture

A partial denture that is cemented to natural teeth or roots which furnish the primary support to the prosthesis

Fixed Prosthesis

A restoration or replacement which is attached by a cementing medium to natural teeth, roots and implants

Pontic

It is a suspended member of a fixed partial denture that replaces the lost natural tooth, restores function and occupies the space of the missing tooth

Abutment

A tooth, a portion of a tooth or that portion of an implant which used for the support of a fixed or removable prosthesis

Ante's law

It has been stated in the glossary as follows, in fixed partial denture prosthodontics for the observation that the combined pericemental area of all the abutment teeth supporting a fixed partial denture should be equal to or greater in pericemental area than the tooth or teeth being replaced; as formulated for removable partial prosthodontics, the combined pericemental area of the abutment teeth plus the mucosa area of the denture base should be equal to or greater than the pericemental area of the missing teeth

Occlusion

The static relationship between the incising and masticating surfaces of the maxillary or mandibular teeth or tooth analogues

Centric Occlusion

The occlusion of opposing teeth when the mandible is at centric relation. This may or may not coincide with the maximum intercuspation

Maximum Intercuspation

The complete intercuspation of the opposing teeth independent of condylar position

Components of Occlusion

The various elements that are involved in occlusion, such as the temporomandibular joints, the associated neuromusculature, teeth, their contacting surfaces alongwith investing tissues and/or the denture supporting structures

Eccentric Occlusion

An occlusion other than centric occlusion

Occlusion Plane

The intentional alteration of the occlusal surfaces of teeth to change their form. The average plane established by the incisal and occlusal surfaces of the teeth

Remounting the Dentures

Any method used to relate restorations to an articulator for the analysis and/or to assist in the development of a plan for occlusal equilibration or reshaping

Abutments

Abutment is the super structure part of the implant, which resembles a prepared tooth, and is designed to be screwed into the implant body. It is the primary component, which provides retention to the prosthesis (fixed partial denture)

Impression Posts

It is a part of the implant that facilitates the transfer of the intraoral location (of the implant or abutment) to a similar position on the cast

Secondary Retention

Retention obtained by retentive features like pins, boxes and grooves, etc. is known as secondary retention. The ability of the restoration to withstand destruction due to external forces is known as structural durability

Chamfer

This finish line possesses a curved slope from the axial wall till the margin

Shoulder

This finish line has a gingival finish wall perpendicular to the axial surfaces of the teeth. If the marginal wall is at 120° to the axial walls, then it is termed a sloping shoulder

Fixed Movable Partial Dentures

A fixed partial denture having one or more non-rigid connectors

Ceramic

It is the most ideal veneering material when used with metal substructure or in all ceramic restorations

Acrylic

Tooth colored acrylic can be used with metallic restorations as a veneer. They are not considered as a permanent material due to poor wear resistance. Recent advances include use of indirect composite resins as veneer materials

Ground Electrode

It is used to complete the electrical circuit as well as helps to stabilise the electrical flow within the patient's body (electrical accidents may occur to the patient if a single electrode is used). It is also known as ground plate, indifferent plate, indifferent electrode, neutral electrode, dispersive electrode, passive electrode and patient return. An electrosurgical unit has an active electrode (A) and ground electrode (B)

Direct Composite Provisional Restoration

This is a new type of resin based provisional restoration for e.g: Bis-acryl composite. This material exibits less heat and curing shrinkage. Hence, it can be fabricated using direct technique intra-orally

Die

A die is a positive replica of the individual prepared tooth on which the margins of the wax patterns are finished. These are individual tooth replicas prepared for easier handling during wax pattern fabrication and finishing of inaccessible areas of the cast

Ceramic/Acrylic Veneering

The ceramic or acrylic veneers in metal resin or metal ceramic restorations are usually added after soldering. These veneers are added onto the cutback area provided in the cast framework

Ceramic Veneering

Ceramic veneering is done in three steps namely preparation of the metal surface, porcelain application and porcelain firing

Cementation

The process of attaching parts by means of a cement

Maxillofacial Prosthodontia

It is the art and science of functional or cosmetic reconstruction by means of non-living substitutes for those regions in the maxilla, mandible and face that are missing or defective because of surgical intervention, trauma, pathology and developmental or congenital malformation. Patients with maxillary defects will have difficulties in mastication, speech and deglutition. The aim of a maxillofacial prosthesis should be to restore the normal physiological function in these patients

Cleft lip and Cleft Palate

Cleft lip occurs due to improper fusion between the fronto-nasal and maxillary process. If this occurs on one side, it leads to a unilateral cleft. If it occurs on both sides, it leads to a bilateral cleft while in Mohr's syndrome, a median (midline) cleft lip is seen

Types of Maxillofacial Injuries

Maxillofacial trauma can be grossly grouped as follows: Fracture of the hard tissues including cranial fractures, orbital fractures, nasal fractures and jaw fractures. Soft tissue injuries involving the temporomandibular joint and other soft tissues adjacent to the trauma site

Implant

In maxillofacial prosthetics, implant is employed as primary retentive structure. Their use may vary from single tooth replacements to extra-oral implants that are used to retain extraoral prosthesis

Obturator

A prosthesis used to close a congenital or acquired tissue opening, primarily of the hard palate and/or contiguous alveolar structures. Prosthetic restoration of the defect often includes use of a surgical obturator, interim obturator, and definitive obturator

Interim Obturators

A prosthesis that is made several weeks or months following the surgical resection of a portion of one or both maxillae. It frequently includes replacement of teeth in the defect area. This prosthesis, when used, replaces the surgical obturator that is placed immediately following the resection and may be subsequently replaced with a definitive obturator

Definitive Obturators

A prosthesis that artificially replaces part or all of the maxilla and the associated teeth lost due to surgery or trauma

Treatment Prosthesis

A prosthetic appliance used for the purpose of treating or conditioning the tissues that are called on to support and retain it

Radiation Carrier

A device used to administer radiation to confined areas by means of capsules, beads, or needles of radiation emitting materials such as radium or cesium. Its function is to hold the radiation source securely in the same position during the entire period of treatment

Acrylic Resin

These materials are preferred for restoring defects that require minimal movement like ocular prosthesis

Acrylic Copolymers

These are plasticized methyl methacrylate polymers with elastic properties. They get tacky leading to the collection of dust and stains, possess poor edge strength, poor durability and degrade under sunlight. Therefore, uncommonly used

Poly Vinyl Chloride and Copolymers

It is a hard, clear, tasteless and odourless resin. It was extensively used in the beginning but its use decreased due to various factors like excessive shrinkage, long processing time, discolouration and hardening of the margins due to plasticizer migration and loss. It absorbs sebaceous secretions and tend to get soiled due to their tackiness

Chlorinated Polyethylene

It is a new material for which clinical trials have just been initiated. It has been first tested by Louis and Castleberry and is found to be similar to polyvinyl chloride. Its disadvantage is that it requires metal moulds for processing

Polyurethane Elastomers

These are elastomers with urethane linkages and are known as polyurethanes. The urethane linkages are formed by combination of one isocyanate group with a hydroxy group. These materials have excellent properties like elasticity without compromised edge strength (this helps to thin the material at the margins). They can be used to restore defects with mobile tissue beds. Their disadvantages include the moisture sensitivity during processing and poor colour stability

Silicones

It is the most commonly used material for facial restoration but properties like poor tear strength and life-less appearance have limited them from universal acceptance

Polyphosphazines

It is a newer material under research. Modifications are required in the commercially available products to be used in maxillofacial prosthetics

Adhesives

Adhesive systems used to retain a maxillofacial prosthesis are classified based on their mode of application. Example: Double sided tapes (most commonly used), pastes, liquid emulsions and spray-ons

Metal

Metal implants are used to obtain bone anchorage for a prosthesis. Implant metals used are mostly titanium alloys. Metal may also be used to make denture bases. Base metal alloys are used for denture base fabrication

Implant

A graft or insert set firmly or deeply into or onto the alveolar process that may be prepared for its insertion

Dental Implant

A substance that is placed into the jaw to support a crown or fixed or removable denture

Abutment

It is the part of the implant, which resembles a prepared tooth and is designed to be screwed into the implant body. It is the primary component which provides retention to the prosthesis (fixed partial denture)

Impression Posts

It is a small stem that facilitates the transfer of the intra oral location (of the implant or abutment) to a similar position on the cast. They are placed over the implant body during impression making

Stent

Eponym, for a device used in conjunction with a surgical procedure to keep a skin graft in place; often modified with acrylic resin or dental modelling impression compound that was previously termed Stent's mass. It also refers to any device or mold used to hold a skin graft in place or provide support for anastomosed structures

Surgical Stent

An appliance named for the dentist who first described its use, Charles R. Stent. It is used to apply pressure to soft tissues to facilitate healing and prevent cicatrisation or collapse

Ceramics

These are inorganic, non-metallic and nonpolymeric materials manufactured by compacting and sintering the different components at high temperatures

PROSTHODONTICS

Classifications

Types of Mandibular Movements

Mandibular movements can be classified as follows:
- Based on the dimension involved in the movement
  - Rotation around the transverse or hinge axis
  - Rotation around the anteroposterior or sagittal axis
  - Rotation around the vertical axis
  - Translation in time.
- Based on the type of movement.
  - Hinge movement.
  - Protrusive movement
  - Retrusive movement
  - Lateral movement
    - Lateral rotation or laterotrusion (Right and left lateral movement).
    - Lateral translation or Bennett movement
      - Immediate side shift
      - Precurrent side shift
      - Progressive side shift
- Based on the extent of movement
  - Border movements

- Extreme movements in the horizontal plane
- Extreme movements in the sagittal plane
- Extreme movements in the coronal plane
- Envelope of motion
- Intra-border movements.
  - Functional movements
    - Chewing cycle
    - Swallowing
    - Yawning
    - Speech
- Para-functional movements
  - Clenching
  - Bruxism
  - Other habitual movements.

Types of Face-bows

Face-bows can be classified as follows:
- Arbitrary face-bow
  - Facia type.
  - Earpiece type
  - Hanau face-bow (Spring bow)
  - Slidematic (Denar)
  - Twirl bow
  - Whipmix
- Kinematic or hinge bow

Types of Balanced Occlusion

Occlusal balance or balanced occlusion can be classified as follows:
- Unilateral balanced occlusion
- Bilateral balanced occlusion
- Protrusive balanced occlusion
- Lateral balanced occlusion

Types of Direct Retainers

Direct retainers are broadly classified as:
- Extracoronal direct retainers (Clasps):
  - Manufactured retainers (Dalbo)
  - Custom-made retainers:
    - Occlusally approaching (Circumferential or Aker's clasp)
    - Gingivally approaching (Bar or Roach's clasp)
- Intracoronal direct retainers (Attachments):
  - Internal attachment
  - External attachment
  - Stud attachment
  - Bar attachment
  - Special attachment

Types of spruing

Spruing can be broadly classified based on the number of sprues used as follows:
- Single spruing
- Multiple spruing (used when the pattern is too long)

Types of Temporary Partial dentures

Three types of temporary partial dentures are as follows:
- Transitional partial denture.
- Interim partial denture.
- Treatment partial denture.

Type of Connectors

Connector in a fixed partial denture can be defined as: The portion of a fixed partial denture that unites the retainer(s) and pontic(s).
- Connectors can be broadly classified as:

- Rigid connectors
- Non-rigid connectors
  - Tenon-Mortise connectors
  - Loop connectors
  - Split pontic connectors
  - Cross pin and wing connectors

Types of Dies

Based on the design, die systems can be classified into:
- Working cast with separate die system
- Working cast with removable die system.

Three commonly used removable die systems are:
- Dowel pin system
  - Straight
  - Curved
- Di-lok tray system
- Pindex system
- Accutrac system

Types of Maxillary Defects

Maxillary defects can be broadly classified as follows:
- Congenital
  - Cleft lip
  - Cleft palate
- Acquired
  - Total maxillectomy
  - Partial maxillectomy

Types of Obturators

Obturators can be classified:
- Based on the phase of treatment:
  - Surgical obturators
    - Immediate obturators
    - Delayed obturators

- Interium obturators.
- Definitive obturators
- Based on the material used:
  - Metal Obturators
  - Resin obturators
  - Silicon obturators
- Based on the Area of Restoration.
  - Polatal obturators
  - Meatel obturators

Classification of FPD

- Class: A class identifies the location of the edentulous space

Class I	Posterior edentulous spaces. One or more of the posterior teeth (premolars and molars) are missing.
Class II	Anterior edentulous spaces. One or more of the anterior teeth (incisors and canines) are missing.
Class III	Antero-posterior edentulous spaces. Edentulous spaces involving both the anterior and posterior regions, i.e. some anterior and posterior teeth are missing.

- Division: A division gives information about the teeth present adjacent to the edentulous space that are capable of taking support.

Division I	Cantilever Fixed Partial Dentures. Abutments present only on one side of the edentulous space are capable of taking support.
Division II	Conventional Fixed Partial Dentures. Abutments that are capable of taking up occlusal load are present on both sides of the edentulous space.
Division III	Pier abutments. A tooth is surrounded by an edentulous space on either side.

- Sub-Division: A sub-division denotes the status of the tooth that is to be used as an abutment.

Sub-division I	Ideal abutments. Healthy teeth, which provide good support
Sub-division II	Tilted abutments. Either the design of the prosthesis should be modified or the tilt of the abutment should be corrected
Sub-division III	Periodontally weak abutment. This abutment cannot take up occlusal load as effectively as healthy abutment
Sub-division IV	Extensively damaged abutment. The abutment has good bone support but require extensive restoration. e.g. inlay, onlay and dowel core
Sub-division V	Implant abutment. The abutment is an implant and the design of the prosthesis should be modified accordingly

- Each sub-division can be further grouped into :
  - A: The support for one side of the edentulous space is taken from a single abutment.
  - B: The support for one side of the edentulous space is taken from more than one abutment tooth.

Other systems of classfication:

- Depending on the type of connector:
  - Fixed fixed partial denture
  - Fixed movable partial denture
  - Removable fixed partial denture
- Type of material used:
  - All metal crowns
  - Metal ceramic crowns
  - All ceramic crowns
  - All acrylic crowns
  - Ceramic veneer

- Acrylic veneer
- Length of the span:
  - Short span bridges
  - Long span bridges
- Duration of use:
  - Permanent fixed partial dentures
  - Long span bridges
    - Interim prosthesis
    - Periodontally weak abutment (Maryland bridge)
    - Splints
- Type of abutment:
  - Normal/ideal abutment
  - Cantilever abutment
  - Pier abutment
  - Mesially tilted abutment
    - Mesial half crown
    - Telescopic crown
- Endodontically treated abutment (depending on the amount of remaining tooth structure)
  - Core: plastic core materials
    - Amalgam
    - Composite
    - Glass-Ionomer cements
    - Pin-retained amalgam
  - Post core restorations
    - Custom-made posts
    - Prefabricated posts
  - Periodontally weak teeth
    - Resin bonded bridges
    - Fiber reinforced bridges
    - Splints
  - Implant abutments

- Bridges which require minimal preparation
  - Micro-retention
  - Macro-retention

Classification of pontics

- Mucosal Contact: Based on the amount of mucosal contact, pontics can be classified as:
  - With mucosal contact
    - Saddle Pontic
    - Ridge Lap Pontic
    - Modified Ridge Lap Pontic
    - Ovate Pontic
  - Without mucosal contact
    - Bullet Pontic
    - Hygienic or Sanitary Pontic
- Type of Material Used: Based on the type of material used, pontics can be classified as:
  - Metal and Porcelain Veneered Pontic
  - Metal and Resin Veneered Pontic
  - All Metal Pontic
  - All ceramic pontic
- Method of Fabrication: Based on the method of fabrication, pontics can be classified as:
  - Custom made pontic
  - Prefabricated pontic
    - Trupontic
    - Interchangeable facing
    - Sanitary Pontic
    - Pin-facing Pontic
    - Modified Pin-facing Pontic
    - Reverse Pin-facing Pontic
    - Harmony Pontic
    - Porcelain Fused to Metal Pontic
  - Prefabricated Custom Modified Pontic

Classification of occlusal arrangements

Characteristics	Cusp-Fossa	Cusp-Marginal Ridge
Location of contact on opposing side	Occlusal fossa only	Marginal ridge and occlusal fossa
Relation with opposing tooth (teeth)	Tooth-to-tooth	Tooth-to two teeth
Advantages	Occlusal forces are directed parallel to the long axis	Most natural type of occlusion (seen in 95% adults). Can be used for single tooth restorations
Disadvantages	It can be used only when several contacting teeth and the teeth opposing them are to be restored	Food impaction and displacement of teeth may arise if the functional cusps wedge into a lingual embrasure
Application	Full mouth reconstruction	Most cast restorations done in daily practice

Classification of Splints

- Based on the extent of the prosthesis across the midline, fixed partial denture splints can be classified as:
  - Unilateral splints
  - Bilateral or cross-arch splints
- Based on the duration of use, fixed partial denture splints can be classified into:
  - Temporary or provisional splints
  - Permanent splints
  - Full rectified, filtered current.

Classification of Maxillofacial Prostheses

A wide variety of maxillofacial prostheses are being fabricated in practice. Based on the location, use, and area of restoration, maxillofacial prostheses can be classified as follows:

- Intraoral
- Maxillary
  - Congenital
    - Cleft lip
    - Cleft palate
  - Acquired
    - Total maxillectomy
      - Complete dentures
      - Partial dentures
      - Obturators
      - Speech aids
      - Implants
    - For partial maxillectomy
      - Complete dentures
      - Partial dentures
- Mandibular
  - Congenital
    - Cleft lip
    - Early feeding devices
    - Surgical
    - Orthodontic
    - Prosthodontic
    - Fixed partial dentures
    - Complete dentures
    - Implants
  - Acquired
    - Complete dentures
    - Partial dentures

- Flange prosthesis
- Mandibular exercisers
- Implants
- Extraoral
  - Auricular prosthesis
  - Ocular prosthesis
  - Orbital prosthesis
  - Nasal prosthesis
  - Composite prosthesis
  - Lip and cheek prosthesis
- Treatment supplements
- Radiotherapy supplements
  - Stents
  - Splints
  - Shields
  - Carriers
  - Positioners
  - Radiation appliances
- Surgical supplements
  - Prosthetic dressings
  - Surgical splints
  - Surgical obturators
- Chemotherapeutic supplements

Classification of Clefts

Classification based on the extent of the defect:
- Clefts can be classified into three types under this category,

Class I	Cleft lip with cleft alveolus (primary palate)
Class II	Cleft of hard and soft palate (secondary palate)
Class III	Combination of I and II

- Veau's Classification of Cleft Palate: Veau (1922) classified cleft palate into four types:

Class I	Cleft involving the soft palate. It can also be a submucous cleft, which appears normal
Class II	A midline cleft involving the bone, present only on the posterior part of the palate
Class III	A unilateral cleft extending along the mid-palatine suture and a suture between premaxilla and palatine shelf
Class IV	A unilateral cleft extending along the mid-palatine suture and both the sutures

PROSTHODONTICS

Viva-Voce

1. **A Glossary of prosthodontics terms is made by**

   Ans. The Federation of Prosthodontic Organization

2. **Example of prosthesis are**

   Ans. A denture, an abturator, fixed denture and a crown

3. **Partial denture is supported by**

   Ans. Dual support soft tissue and tooth support

4. **An interim denture is**

   Ans. Dental prosthesis to be used for a short period for mastication and phonetics

5. **An abutment is**

   Ans. The portion of a tooth and portion of an implant that serves as support

6. **In Kennedy-Applegate classification the deciding factor is**

   Ans. Missing of most posterior tooth

7. Kennedy class III classification is

Ans. Unilateral edentulous area with natural teeth both anterior and posterior to it

8. Kennedy-Applegate class VI classification is

Ans. An edentulous situation in which the teeth anterior to the space are capable of total support of the required prosthesis

9. The sequence of classification system depends on

Ans. The frequency of occurence and the principles of design

10. In Kennedy's classification, the most common arch is

Ans. Class I

11. Totally tooth supported prosthesis is

Ans. Class III partial denture

12. An acceptable method of classification

Ans. It should be universally acceptable and permit differentiation between tooth supported and tissue supported partial denture. It should serve as a guide to the type of design to be used

13. The conditions not considered in Kennedy's classification are

Ans. When third molar is absent, it should not to be replaced. If a second molar is missing, it is even not to be replaced

14. Patient comes with only the first molar in the lower arch, the classification is

Ans. Class-I Mod-1

15. Kennedy-Applegate classification of partially edentulous arch does not allow consideration of

Ans. Length of the edentulous spaces

16. In palatal major connector relief should always be given for

Ans. Palatal torus

17 The main advantage of palatal plate major connectors is

Ans. Thin metal plate

18. The main aim of providing occlusal rests is

Ans. To distribute occlusal loads to the abutment teeth and to resist vertical force of occlusion

19. The retentive tip should be placed in which area of crown?

Ans. Cervical 1/3rd

20. The most suitable material for taking impression of a partial edentulous mouth is

Ans. Elastomers

21. Guiding planes prepared on enamel surfaces should be

Ans. Flat

22. The seat for occlusal rest on abutment should be

Ans. On the marginal ridge at 90 degrees to the long axis of the abutment

23. The main function of reciprocal clasp arm is

Ans. To counteract the forces transmitted by the retentive arm

24. **The process by which one part of the removable partial denture opposes the action of retainer in function is called?**

Ans. Reciprocation

25. **Complete crowns on a tilted abutment tooth for clasp retained removable partial denture serves mainly**

Ans. To provide favourable contour of the abutment

26. **In removable partial denture indirect retainers should be placed**

Ans. On opposite side of the fulcrum line of the denture base and much away from the direct retainer

27. **The main function of the indirect retainer is to**

Ans. Minimise the movement of denture away from the supporting tissue

28. **One of the important functions of the clasp in removable partial denture is**

Ans. To prevent the dislodgement of the denture

29. **Major connector of removable partial denture should be**

Ans. Rigid to connect bilateral components of removable partial denture

30. **The ideal shape of the occlusal rest seat on the posterior teeth is**

Ans. Spoon or saucer shaped

31. **The cause of greatest damage by a partial denture is**

Ans. Flexibility of the major connector

32. The major connector should never terminate on gingival tissues because

Ans. The marginal gingiva is highly vascular and susceptible to injury from pressure

33. Beading should have a depth and width of approximately

Ans. 0.5–1 mm

34. Auxiliary rests are

Ans. Indirect retainer

35. For a distal extension partial denture, the occlusal rest seat should be

Ans. Shallow and saucer shaped

36. The outline form of an occlusal rest should be

Ans. Triangular

37. Location of the incisal rest from the proximal incisal angle of the tooth is approximately

Ans. 1.5–2 mm

38. The rest seat for a lingual rest is

Ans. V-shaped

39. Incisal rests are most frequently used on

Ans. Mandibular canine

40. Lingual rests are most frequently used on

Ans. Maxillary canine

41. The height of contour is

Ans. A line at which occlusally sloping surfaces meet cervically sloping surfaces

42. The clasp except the retentive clasp terminal is always located

Ans. Occlusal to the height of contour

43. Retentive clasp arm is divided into

Ans. Three parts

44. Clasp must be designed to encircle

Ans. 200 degrees of the abutment tooth

45. The ring clasp should not be considered on a mandibular molar due to

Ans. Attachment of buccinators muscle close to the tooth

46. Bar clasp have

Ans. Push type retention

47. Modified 'T' clasp is basically a

Ans. T clasp with no nonretentive finger

48. The most effective location of an indirect retainer is

Ans. A line projected at right angles from the fulcrum line and ending in a tooth

49. The teeth which are not normally selected to support indirect retainers are?

Ans. Incisors

50. Effectiveness of indirect retainer is influenced by

Ans. Position in rest seat

51. Facing is a

Ans. Thin veneer of tooth coloured porcelain or acrylic resin attached to a metal backing or natural tooth

Viva-Voce

52. Distance between maxillary major connector and tooth tissue junction is

Ans. 6 mm

53. Mandibular major connector should be placed from gingival crest to at least

Ans. 4 mm

54. Minimum thickness of occlusal rest if chrome alloy is used

Ans. 1 mm

55. What is the minimum thickness of occlusal rest if gold is used?

Ans. 1 5 mm

56. Length of maxillary central incisor is

Ans. Hairline-chin distance/16

57. Most common cause associated with gagging in maxillary partial denture is

Ans. Lingual bar

58. Designing of removable partial denture starts

Ans. When taking jaw relation after casts are ready

59. Terminal end of the retentive arm should be placed at which part of the crown?

Ans. Cervical third

60. The most important consideration in designing bilateral lower distal extension removable partial denture replacing only molars is

Ans. Load distribution

61. Class I, II and IV removable partial dentures are subjected to greater stresses because of

Ans. Poor source of support

62. Average closing force of the natural teeth is

Ans. 53.58 kg per sq cm (300 pounds per square inch)

63. Triangular or tripod configuration is ideal for

Ans. Class II arch

64. Artificial dentures absorb more stress in case of

Ans. Large, broad and well formed ridge

65. The types of clasping configuration required for a class I partially edentulous arches are

Ans. Bilateral configuration

66. Periodontally weakened teeth can be stabilized against horizontal forces by

Ans. A removable partial denture

67. Maxillary bilateral distal extension dentures need

Ans. Simultaneous working and balancing side contact

68. For tooth supported partial dentures, denture base flange is kept

Ans. Just short of reflection of soft tissue

69. Minimum thickness of periphery of the denture base on the distal extension edentulous ridge is

Ans. 2 mm

70. Who described the phenomenon of Realiff factor?

Ans. Hanau

71. The function of the scriber in a surveyor

Ans. Marks the greatest convexity of the tooth surface

72. The best path of insertion of a removable partial denture is

Ans. Perpendicular to occlusal plane

73. Ney surveyor and Wills surveyor are differentiated on account of

Ans. Surveying arm

74. The height of contour on the tooth is formed by

Ans. Analyzing rod

75. Which part of retentive clasp arm is placed gingival to survey line?

Ans. Terminal one-third

76. Retentive undercuts must be present on the abutment teeth at the

Ans. Horizontal tilt

77. The most desired location that is needed for Ideal undercut

Ans. 0.03937 mm (0.010 inch)

78. What is given least priority if esthetics is the patient's primary concern?

Ans. Removable partial dentures

79. In patients with a large palatal torus, the choice of major connector is

Ans. Anteroposterior palatal bar

80. In case of flat or flabby ridges or shallow vault, the very useful major connector is

Ans. Complete palate

81. Anterior palatal strap should be

Ans. As far anteriorly as possible

82. Beading is never used in mandibular major connectors due to

Ans. The need for relief required under all mandibular major connectors

83. The location of the lingual bar in the patient's mouth should be

Ans. Inferior

84. Minimum vertical space between active tissues of floor of mouth and gingival of teeth for lingual major connector is

Ans. 8 mm

85. The superior border of the lingual bar should lie

Ans. At least 4 mm below the gingival margin

86. Ideal clasp position for retentive clasp is in

Ans. Gingival third

87. Most easily compromised factor in selection of path of insertion is

Ans. Guiding planes

88. A class I prosthesis usually requires how many retentive clasp arms?

Ans. Two

89. In removable partial denture, quadrilateral positioning of direct retainer is ideal for

Ans. Class III prosthesis

90. What should be the minimum occlusogingival height of lingual bar for proper rigidity?

Ans. 5 mm

91. Width of the preparation for embrasure clasp is

Ans. 1.5–2.0 mm

92. What is the depth of the preparation for embrasure clasp?

Ans. 1–1.5 mm

93. The fixed splint provide increased resistance by

Ans. Anteroposterior forces

94. What provides cross-arch stabilization to forces operating in a buccolingual direction?

Ans. Removable partial denture

95. Material of choice for swing-lock framework is

Ans. Chrome alloy

96. Most important indication for use of overdenture abutment is

Ans. To provide support for long-span anterior edentulous areas

97. How much size of the tooth shoud be reduced in case of overdenture abutment, above the proximal gingival margin?

Ans. 2–3 mm

98. In which types of defect of the maxilla, retention is most easily attained?

Ans. Class II

99. Most versatile maxillary major connector is

Ans. Palatal starp

100. Faciolingual width of artificial teeth used to replace the missing posterior teeth should be

Ans. 2/3rd of the natural teeth

101. Depth of adequate incisal rest on tooth is

Ans. 1.5 mm

102. The enclosed angle formed by inclination of the floor of the rest and the vertical projection of the proximal surface of the tooth must be

Ans. Less than 90 degrees

103. Denture given when some or all of the remaining teeth are beyond the point of restoration but immediate extraction is not indicated for physiologic or psychological reason is

Ans. Transitional denture

104. Most critical reduction of overdenture abutment is on

Ans. Labial side

105. The taper of preparation of overdenture abutment tooth from the labiogingival margin to the center of the tooth must be

Ans. 25°–30°

106. The tapering of proximal and lingual reduction of overdenture abutment tooth makes

Ans. 10°–15°

107. Buccal and lingual surface of abutment tooth of unilateral removable partial denture is

Ans. Parallel

108. Plastic scalers are used in removing calculus from

Ans. Implant crown

109. The most commonly used impression material for diagnostic casts of removable partial denture is

Ans. Irreversible hydrocolloid

110. Most suitable impression material for clasp retainer removable partial denture is

Ans. Alginate

111. Which impression technique is needed in class I and class II removable partial denture prosthesis?

Ans. Selective pressure technique

112. Impression material of choice for the swing-lock denture is

Ans. Alginate

113. The main drawback of using methacryloyloxyethy trimellitate anhydride is that

Ans. It is more difficult to pack the acrylic resin dough

114. The tissue stop is made by removing approximately

Ans. 2 square mm of the relief wax

115. Internal finish line is developed as master cast is relieved

Ans. Before duplication

116. The angle the finish line forms with the major connector should be

Ans. Less than 90 degrees

117. Minimum width of finish line of removable partial denture is

Ans. 1 mm

118. What is the minimum distance between finish line and abutment teeth in removable partial denture?

Ans. 1.5–2 mm

119. Most common relief in partial denture is associated with

Ans. Denture base

120. Most commonly used alloy for retentive clasp arm is

Ans. Chromium-cobalt-nickel

121. Encirclement of each clasp is

Ans. More than 180 degrees

122. Circumferential clasp is

Ans. Akers clasp

123. Easiest clasp to design and construct is

Ans. Cast circumferential clasp

124. Ring clasp is most often indicated in

Ans. Tipped molars

125. Which type of contacts are needed in class IV partial denture?

Ans. Light contact in centric occlusion and no contact in eccentric position

126. Maxillary unilateral distal extension dentures needed

Ans. Working side contact only

127. Simple hinge articulators are frequently indicated for

Ans. Class III partial edentulous state

128. Semiadjustable articulator is mostly indicated for

Ans. Class I partial edentulous state and complete denture cases

129. Which gauge wire is used for retentive clasp in interim partial denture?

Ans. 0.1574 mm (0.040 inch)

130. First component of the interim partial denture to be formed is

Ans. Retentive clasp

131. The role of lingual plate is

Ans. A horizontal stability to a removable partial denture and prevent excessive lateral forces on the teeth when used in splint

132. In which type of defect of the maxilla retention is most easily attained?

Ans. Class II

133. How many times patients should clean their removable partial denture?

Ans. After every meal

134. Time intervals between examinations in case of partial denture should not normally exceed

Ans. Twelve months

135. Minimum width of ridge needed for biointegrated hydroxyapatite-coated dental implants is

Ans. 5 mm

136. Minimum bone height of ridge needed for biointegrated hydroxyapatite-coated dental implant is

Ans. 8 mm

137. Who utilized titanium first time as the implant material?

Ans. Brane Mark

138. How much space is needed between implant and inferior alveolar canal?

Ans. 2 mm

139. Which is the most reliable and useful diagnostic tool for examining the periodontium?

Ans. Periodontal probe

140. Pulp vitality can be tested by

Ans. Pulp tester, thermal stimulation and preparing a test cavity

141. What is used to control setting rate in alginate?

Ans. Trisodium phosphate

Viva-Voce

142. Which impression material does not undergoe dimensional changes, if not poured immediately ?

Ans. Alginate

143. After removing from the mouth, the alginate impression should be poured within

Ans. 15 minutes

144. What is the change in setting expansion of gypsum cast, if immersed in water?

Ans. Setting expansion increases

145. Name one non-arcon articulator.

Ans. Dentatus

146. Which articulator is fully adjustable?

Ans. Denar D5-A

147. Example of semiadjustable articulators are

Ans. Dentatus, Whip mix and Hanau 96 H2O

148. Total number of plates required in pantographic recording are

Ans. 6 plates

149. Name one plastic material.

Ans. Silver amalgam

150. Prosthesis in which only one side of pontic is attached to a retainer is called as?

Ans. Cantilever fixed partial denture

151. What is an ideal abutment?

Ans. Unrestored caries free tooth

152. **The root surface area of the abutment should be greater than the root surface area of the tooth to be replaced. This law is known as**

Ans. Ante's law

153. **The average root surface area of the maxillary permanent 1st molar is**

Ans. 433 mm^2

154. **Which tooth provides better support in fixed partial denture?**

Ans. A molar with divergent roots

155. **The deflection of a fixed partial denture is proportional to the**

Ans. Cube of the length of span

156. **The long span fixed partial denture should be fabricated by a material having**

Ans. High strength and high rigidity

157. **When replacing the four maxillary incisors with fixed partial denture, the abutment usually used are**

Ans. Both canines and first premolars only

158. **Which gingival margins is less conservative than other gingival margins?**

Ans. Shoulder

159. **Which gingival margins is occasionally indicated on tilted teeth?**

Ans. Chisel edge

160. **Which gingival margins is usually indicated on facial margins of metal ceramic crowns?**

Ans. Shoulder

161. The recommended convergence between opposing walls is

Ans. 6 degrees

162. Which are accessory means of retention form of the restoration?

Ans. Grooves, boxe, pinholes and all of the above

163. Which gold alloys are usually used for fabrication of fixed partial denture?

Ans. Type III and Type IV

164. What are the indications for all metal cast crown?

Ans. Badly damaged posterior teeth, endodontically treated teeth correction of occlusal plane

165. Which restoration has greater retention as compared to others?

Ans. All metal complete cast crown

166. Which is a contraindication for all metal cast crown?

Ans. Esthetics

167. The recommended clearance of centric cusps in all cast metal crown is

Ans. 1.5 mm

168. The thickness of the metal allowed by chamfer margin at the margin in all cast metal crown is approximately

Ans. 0.5 mm

169. During tooth preparation for a complete cast crown, the functional cusp bevel is placed at how many degrees to long axis of the tooth?

Ans. 45°

170. Which factor is not a contraindication for metal-ceramic crown?

Ans. Esthetics

171. The recommended incisal reduction for metal-ceramic crown is

Ans. 2 mm

172. What is an advantage of metal ceramic crown?

Ans. Superior esthetics as compared to gold restorations

173. The recommended clearance in intercuspal positions and all excursions in metal ceramic crown is

Ans. 1.5–2.0 mm

174. Which gingival margin is recommended for lingual margin of metal ceramic crown?

Ans. Chamfer

175. Which restoration technique is less retentive as compared to others?

Ans. Inlay and onlay

176. Which partial veneer crowns is usually not used in posterior teeth?

Ans. Pinledge

177. Which surface of tooth is not involved in three-quarter crown preparation?

Ans. Facial surface

178. Inlay is

Ans. An intracoronal restoration which does not cover all the cusps

Viva-Voce 61

179. Which type of crown does not involve the mesial half of the buccal surface?

Ans. Seven-eighth crown

180. When Pinledge preparation is used to re-establish anterior guidance than it involves

Ans. Lingual surface of the tooth

181. Which retainer is most conservative of tooth structure?

Ans. Pinledge

182. The recommended gingival margin in porcelain jacket crown is

Ans. Shoulder on all surfaces of tooth

183. The recommended width of shoulder in porcelain jacket crown is

Ans. 1.0 mm circumferentially

184. The optimal cavosurface angle in all ceramic crown is

Ans. 90°

185. The recommended incisal reduction for the porcelain jacket crown is

Ans. 1.5 mm

186. In porcelain jacket crown, centric contacts

Ans. Are confined to incisal third of the lingual surface

187. Which surface of the tooth is more reduced in metal ceramic crown as compared to complete ceramic crown?

Ans. Facial surface

188. Which etchant is used in bonding of porcelain to tooth?

Ans. Hydrofluoric acid

189. The ceramic inlays and onlays are contraindicated in patients with

Ans. Poor oral hygiene, active caries and excessive occlusal loading such as people suffering from bruxism

190. Which porcelain is less abrasive?

Ans. Castable glass-ceramic

191. Give a characteristic feature of working cast?

Ans. It must be free from voids

192. What is the critical characteristic of cast and die materials?

Ans. Resistance to abrasion and dimensional accuracy

193. Which type of gypsum products is high strength dental stone?

Ans. Type IV

194. If the soaking of gypsum cast is required in water, it should be soaked in water saturated with

Ans. Plaster slurry

195. Which impression materials are not compatible with resin dies?

Ans. Polysulfide and hydrocolloid

196. Which impression material can be electroplated to form electroplated dies?

Ans. Polysulfide

197. Which die material is recommended in most of the situations?

Ans. Type IV dental stone

198. Practically all wax patterns are made by the

Ans. Indirect technique in the laboratory

199. Most dental castings are made.

Ans. Indirectly by lost wax process

200. The optimum space required between the internal surface of the casting and the prepared surface of the tooth for each wall is

Ans. 20–40 μm

201. What is the main constituent of the inlay casting wax?

Ans. Paraffin wax

202. Which constituent of the inlay casting wax decreases the melting temperature of the wax?

Ans. Candelilla wax

203. According to ADA specification, how much residue of wax can be permitted during the wax burnout procedure?

Ans. 0.1%

204. The inlay casting wax used for making wax pattern in direct technique should be carved, burnished and polished when the temperature reaches

Ans. 37° C

205. What can be used as an occlusal indicator paste?

Ans. Zinc stearate

206. According to ADA specification, which type of waxes is generally used for the indirect fabrication of castings?

Ans. Type II

207. What is not a biological factor for pontic design?

Ans. Rigid (to resist deformation)

208. Which pontics does not contact mucosa of the ridge?

Ans. Sanitary type

209. Which pontic design contacts mucosa of the ridge?

Ans. Ridge lap

210. Which pontic design has only one point contact at the centre of the residual ridge?

Ans. Bullet shaped pontic

211. The modified ridge lap pontic design is usually recommended in

Ans. Maxillary anterior region

212. Which pontic design is usually recommended in mandibular posterior region?

Ans. Sanitary type

213. Which pontic design is most hygienic?

Ans. Sanitary type

214. Porcelain is a

Ans. Brittle material

215. Which material can be kept plaque free easily as compared to others?

Ans. Glazed porcelain

216. In metal-ceramic restorations, during centric and eccentric movements, the occlusal contacts should not fall on

Ans. Metal-ceramic junction

217. Which pontic is needed in situations of high stress?

Ans. All metal pontic

218. Which pontic are contraindicated where esthetics is important?

Ans. All metal pontic

219. The wax pattern should

Ans. Be invested immediately

220. Which sprue is preferred for most castings?

Ans. Wax sprue

221. Which sprue is recommended for molars?

Ans. 10 gauge

222. Which diameter of sprue is recommended for one molar metal-ceramic patterns?

Ans. 2.5 mm diameter

223. Which sprue is recommended for premolars and partial coverage restoration?

Ans. 12 gauge

224. The sprue should be attached to the

Ans. Thickest part of the pattern

225. In posterior teeth, the sprue should be attached to

Ans. Largest noncentric cusp

226. What was earlier used as a ring liner of casting ring?

Ans. Asbestos

227. The angle formed by sprue attached to wax pattern with the axial wall is

Ans. $135°$

228. Which investment is recommended for metal-ceramic frameworks?

Ans. Phosphate bonded investments

229. Which type of casting alloys are hard?

Ans. Type III

230. Which factors increase expansion of gypsum bonded investment?

Ans. Storage at 100% humidity, lower water powder ratio and use of a dry liner

231. The suck back porosity is caused when

Ans. The sprue is too narrow, hot spot is created and mold melt temperature difference is high.

232. In metal ceramic restoration, the ceramic is bounded to metal

Ans. Both by mechanical and chemical bonds

233. The intended metal ceramic junction should be at

Ans. $90°$

234. The minimum thickness of the metal coping in metal-ceramic restoration made up of noble metal alloys is

Ans. 0.3 mm

235. The minimum thickness of metal coping of base metal alloys is

Ans. 0.2 mm

236. The mechanical properties of the metal-ceramic restoration mainly depend on

Ans. Design of the metal framework

227. Which base elements are used to form oxide layer in metal ceramic restoration?

Ans. Tin, indium and iron

238. The fusion temperature of medium fusing porcelain is

Ans. 1090° C-1260° C

239. Feldspar contains oxides of

Ans. Sodium and potassium

240. The absence of crystallization on cooling and solidification is called as

Ans. Vitrification

241. Which oxides are added to original porcelain to mask the color of underlying metal coping?

Ans. Oxides of titanium, oxides of chromium and oxides of chromium and tin

242. The thickness of opaque porcelain should not exceed

Ans. 0.2 mm

243. Collarless crowns have

Ans. Facial margin of porcelain

244. Which techniques are used to fabricate porcelain labial margin in metal ceramic restorations?

Ans. Platinum foil matrix, cyanoacrylate resin and porcelain wax

245. The first ceramic crowns and inlays were made by

Ans. C. H Land

246. Dicor porcelain should be subjected to

Ans. 11 hour firing sequence

247. Leucite contains

Ans. Potassium, aluminium and silicate

248. Ion exchange method on the surface of the ceramic

Ans. Limits crack extension

249. The thickness of the platinum foil used in fabrication of porcelain jacket crown should be

Ans. 0.001 inch

250. The strength of the ceramic in moist environment

Ans. Is decreased

251. The conventional fixed prosthodontics techniques are generally contraindicated in young patients because of

Ans. Inadequate plaque control, participation in sports and large size of the pulps

252. The resin-retained restorations are contraindicated in patients with

Ans. A parafunctional habits, non-existent occlusion and long edentulous span

253. Which tooth abutment is unsuitable as a resin-retained restoration?

Ans. Unrestored tooth

254. Which prosthesis is formed by electrolytic etching is also known as Maryland bridge?

Ans. Resin restained prosthesis

255. What is used for etching in electrolytic etching process for resin retained restoration with beryllium containing alloy?

Ans. 10% sulphuric acid (H_2SO_4)

256. The electrochemical etching for non-beryllium containing resin retained restoration is done with

Ans. Nitric acid + hydrochloric acid

257. A process which involves the use of an intermediate metal whose melting temperature is lower than parent metal is called as?

Ans. Soldering

258. The process in which filler has a melting point above 450^0 C is called as?

Ans. Brazing

259. The recommended soldering gap is

Ans. 0.25 mm

260. Which connector is used to maintain a diastema in the planned fixed prosthesis?

Ans. Loop connector

261. The intermediate abutment in fixed prosthesis is also known as

Ans. Pier abutment

262. The male part of non-rigid connector used in fixed partial denture is also known as

Ans. Tenon

263. Quenching immediately after soldering

Ans. Causes the fixed partial denture to warp

264. One of the disadvantages of the postceramic soldering is

Ans. It is very technical sensitive

265. Which soldering flux is used with gold alloys?

Ans. Borax glass flux

266. The soldering flux formula does not contain

Ans. Iron oxide 35 parts

267. What is used as soldering antiflux?

Ans. Graphite

268. Rouge contains

Ans. Iron oxide

269. Which zones of the flame is used in torch soldering?

Ans. Reducing or neutral zone

270. Infrared soldering is used for

Ans. Preceramic soldered joints

271. The recommended special presolder melts at

Ans. 1110° C-1127° C

272. The adjustment in glazed restoration can be made with

Ans. Fine diamond points

273. A gold casting deficient in proximal contact can be corrected by

Ans. Soldering

274. The "negative space" is the name given to the shape of

Ans. Occlusal embrasures

275. The strength of poly methylmethacrylate resin is

Ans. 1.20th of the metal ceramic alloys

276. In fixed partial denture, what is often site of fracture?

Ans. Connector

277. Overcontoured connector may cause

Ans. Accumulation of plaque, pressure ischemia and gingivitis

278. Which of the following are available in transparent sheets?

Ans. Cellulose acetate and polypropylene

279. Which material used for preformed provisional restoration has the most natural appearance?

Ans. Polycarbonate

280. Which provisional restorations is extensively used on primary teeth?

Ans. Nickel-chromium

281. Which is not an ideal property of the provisional restoration materials?

Ans. Dimensionally unstable during solidification

282. Which is not a biocompatible property of the provisional restorative materials?

Ans. Exothermic

283. The monomer gets vaporized at a temperature near

Ans. 100° C

284. The decomposition of benzoyl peroxide to free radicals in chemically activated resin is catalysed by

Ans. Tertiary amine

285. What is the most commonly used luting agent for provisional restoration?

Ans. Modified zinc-oxide eugenol cement

286. The most commonly used implant is

Ans. Endosteal implant

287. Ideally for an implant placement how much vertical and horizontal bone is required?

Ans. (a) Vertical bone-10 mm, (b) Horizontal bone-6 mm

288. The minimum recommended distance between two adjacent implants is

Ans. 3 mm

289. The minimum distance between apical end of implant and superior aspect of inferior alveolar canal should be

Ans. 2 mm

Viva-Voce

290. The minimum distance between an implant and adjacent tooth should be

Ans. 1 mm

291. The minimum time required for adequate integration of the implant in maxilla should be

Ans. 6 months

292. The minimum amount of bone that should be present between implant and maxillary sinus should be

Ans. 1 mm

293. Which is most ideal site for implant placement?

Ans. Anterior mandible

294. The healing period in mandible required after first stage surgery for implant placement is

Ans. 3 months

295. The required healing time for maxilla after first stage surgery for implant is

Ans. 6 months

296. The minimum amount of bone that should be present between implant and nasal floor is

Ans. 1 mm

297. RPI stands for

Ans. RPI stands for
- Rest.
- Plate (proximal).
- I bar clasp.

298. How long prior to taking an impression should the retraction cord be left in place?

Ans. 5 min

299. Coefficient of thermal expansion of metal-ceramic alloy is

Ans. More than or equal to porcelain but not less than porcelain

300. Titanium casting is done

Ans. Under air pressure and in nitrogen atmosphere

301. The sprue in wax pattern should be placed

Ans. At acute angle

302. Minimal occlusal clearance on centric cusp for cast metal is

Ans. 1.5 mm.

303. Which agent is used as a die hardner?

Ans. Cynoacrylate

304. Important diagnostic tool for achieving accurate implant angulation

Ans. Surgical template

305. Cavosurface margin angulation in chamfer finish line is

Ans. 90° or more than 90°

306. The requirement to increase resistance form of an excessively tapered preparation

Ans. To add groove

307. For a patient with missing canine what type of prosthesis we will prefer?

Ans. Implant retained crown

308. A pier abutment is

Ans. With an edentulous space on both side of the abutment

309. In case, if maxillary canine is missing and we have to make a tooth supported fixed partial denture, abutments will be

Ans. Central incisor, lateral incisor and 1st pre-molar

310. Pivoting movement better resisted by a tooth preparation if

Ans. Diameter is smaller

311. Ideal site for implant placement in a completely edentulous mandible

Ans. Interforaminal region

312. Pontic design that in non-indicated in anterior region

Ans. Spheroidal pontic

313. The posterior tooth that gives a better support is

Ans. Divergent roots

314. To replace a missing canine, the best pontic design is

Ans. Modified ridge lap

315. The most suitable margin design for porcelain crown is

Ans. Shoulder

316. All ceramic crowns are not indicated for young children because

Ans. Pulp horns are wide and high

317. Dental implants are treatment of choice when there is

Ans. Maladaptive denture behaviour

318. The aim of prosthodontics treatment of edentulous patient is developing harmony among

Ans. Esthetics, occlusion, mastication and personality

319. What are the causes of maladaptive denture behaviour?

Ans. Anatomical factor, physiological factor and psychological factor

320. Which is the main function of teeth?

Ans. Mastication of food

321. What is the average surface area available for support of complete denture in edentulous maxilla and mandible respectively?

Ans. 22.96 cm^2 and 12.25 cm^2

322. What is average masticatory force of natural dentition?

Ans. 19.95 kg (44 pounds)

323. In the edentulous state, what is analogous to the periodontal ligament?

Ans. Mucous membrane

324. What is approximately the total time that teeth are subjected to functional forces of mastication and deglutition in 24 hours?

Ans. 1050 second

325. Mastication in a complete denture wearing patient can be improved by

Ans. Bilateral muscle effort

326. What is terminal age of skeletal growth in human?

Ans. 20–25 years

327. Loss of all the natural teeth and reduction of residual ridges cause

Ans. Mandibular prognathism

328. In a complete denture wearer, the ratio of the mean reduction in height of residual ridges in anterior region of mandible and maxilla is about

Ans. 4 1

329. In which condition does the centric relation and centric occlusion coincide?

Ans. Complete denture and single complete denture opposing natural teeth

330. Nutrient intake in conventional complete denture wearers as compared to that in dentate subjects is reduced to about

Ans. 20%

331. Chewing efficiency of an average removable denture wearer as compared to an adult with complete natural dentition is about

Ans. 20%–30%

332. Chewing efficiency of an individual with single complete denture opposing natural teeth as compared to a person with complete dentures in both the arches is about

Ans. Almost same

333. 'Cafe' coronary is

Ans. Sudden accidental death of denture wearing patients in restaurants due to chocking of food in the air or food passage

334. Accumulation of fat in the body leads to

Ans. Decrease in metabolic ate

335. National Cholesterol Education Program (NCEP) of National Heart Blood and Lung Institute (NHBLI) has recommended the intake of saturated fat as

Ans. 8%–10% of total calorie intake

336. NCEP of NHBLI has recommended the intake of polyunsaturated fats as

Ans. Up to 10% of total calorie intake

337. Monounsaturated fats are superior to polyunsaturated fats because they

Ans. Depress low density lipoproteins without lowering high density lipoproteins

338. Protein requirement of older individuals as compared to younger individuals is

Ans. Slightly higher

339. Proteins provide

Ans. 12%–14% of total calories intake

340. Body water is about

Ans. 50% of total muscle mass in the body

341. What is the cause of Bitot spots?

Ans. Accumulation of desquamated epithelial cells at the inner canthus or eyes due to xerophthalmia

342. What can be used as saliva substitute?

Ans. Milk

343. The average need of calcium is

Ans. 1 g/day

344. The recommended daily dose of calcium for men over 65 years of age and for postmenopausal women taking no estrogen is

Ans. 1.5 g/day

345. Which vitamin prevents the growth of malignant epithelial tumors?

Ans. Vitamin A

346. Hypovitaminosis A causes

Ans. Hyperkeratosis of oral epithelium and decreased salivary flow

347. Which vitamin has the sparing action on low levels of estrogen in postmenopausal women?

Ans. Vitamin B-complex

348. Hypervitaminosis D causes

Ans. Calcification of soft tissues

349. Protein requirement of elderly persons above 50 years of age is about

Ans. 0.8 g/kg/day

350. The best source of protein for elderly person is

Ans. Boiled meat and fish

351. An edentulous patient with poor oral and denture hygiene wears ill-fitting dentures for maximum time, and presents a diffuse erythematous zone under denture covered area. He is a tobacco smoker also. The most probable diagnosis is

Ans. Denture stomatitis

352. What is the cause of flabby ridge?

Ans. Excessive load on residual ridges

353. A tumor like growth around the denture borders of an unstable new denture is known as

Ans. Epulis fissuratum

354. Gray necrotic membrane, inflammatory halo and firm and elevated borders are characteristic features of

Ans. Traumatic ulcer

355. What is the cause of traumatic ulcer?

Ans. Over extended flanges and occlusal imbalance

356. The probable cause of oral carcinoma in denture wearer is

Ans. Heavy alcohol or tobacco use

357. In burning mouth syndrome, the oral mucosa in contact with the denture appears

Ans. Normal and healthy

358. Burning mouth syndrome is usually are common in

Ans. Females older than 50 years wearing complete dentures

359. What is the sign of burning mouth syndrome?

Ans. Burning mouth syndrome has no apparent clinical sign

360. The ratio of rate of reduction in height of mandible to that of maxilla in edentulous patients is

Ans. 4 1

361. Requirement of which nutrient declines with age?

Ans. Carbohydrates

362. The immediate post-extraction resorption of alveolar bone is usually completed at about

Ans. 3 months following extraction

363. What is a contraindication of vestibuloplasty?

Ans. Severe prognathism

364. What is indication of vestibuloplasty?

Ans. Obliteration of sulci and hamular notch

365. Mucosal grafts are preferred for vestibuloplasty because they are

Ans. Superior to skin grafts

366. What is the osseointegration time of dental implants in old age?

Ans. 5–6 months

367. What acts as disloadging force on denture?

Ans. Adhesiveness of food

368. What is retentive force of complete denture?

Ans. Force of adhesion

369. For adhesion to work as aid in retention of denture, the necessary parameter in

Ans. Saliva

370. What forms ionic bonds with surface epithelium and acrylic resin during the phenomenon of adhesion of denture?

Ans. Charged glycoproteins of saliva

371. Theoretically, the gravitational force is retentive force for

Ans. Mandibular denture

372. The contraindication of denture adhesive is

Ans. Ill-fitting dentures

373. For making a stable complete denture the artificial teeth must be arranged on

Ans. Neutral zone

374. Which teeth provides stable support for denture?

Ans. Premolar and molar area

375. For better support of complete denture, the area of occlusal table of artificial teeth should be

Ans. Less than that of natural dentition

376. In a complete denture-bearing patient, wrinkles around the modiolus, low visibility of vermilion border of lip and weak and turned in lip indicate

Ans. Low vertical dimension of occlusion

377. Maxillary tuberosities usually become redundant due to combination syndrom which results from?

Ans. Wearing of lower distal extension partial denture opposing upper complete denture

378. In a patient, the soft palate turns downward from the hard palate at an angle of about 45^0, it is termed as

Ans. Adequate relief in the complete denture over the torus

379. A radiograph showing a lesion with gross bone destruction without proliferative response indicates

Ans. Rapid growing lesion

380. Which radiograph is helpful to diagnose a jaw lesion which causes buccal or lingual expansion of jaw bone?

Ans. Occlusal radiograph

381. The most common cause of hyperplastic tissue in the anterior part of maxillary residual ridge is

Ans. Maxillary complete denture occludes against natural mandibular anterior teeth and mandibular distal extension prosthesis

382. Tongue function test normally reveals

Ans. Over extended lingual flanges of lower denture

383. The most common site of epulis-fissuratum is

Ans. Around the borders of ill-fitting dentures

384. The main cause of epulis-fissuratum is

Ans. Chronic irritation from ill-fitting dentures

385. After surgical removal of prominent genial tubercles, the genioglossus muscle is sutured to

Ans. Geniohyoid muscle

386. Which ridge undercut is preferably removed surgically?

Ans. Posterior ridge undercut

387. The most common site of undercut in mandible is

Ans. Incisor region

388. If the upper and lower residual ridges are parallel, than the resultant occlusal forces

Ans. Fall on the ridges perpendicularly and tend to seat the dentures

389. In a denture wearing patient with extremely resorbed mandibular ridge, there is pain and paresthesia of the lower lip. What can be the most probable cause?

Ans. Pressure on the mental nerve by denture base

390. The most common site of bony exostosis is

Ans. Buccal side of posterior maxilla

391. Name one stress-bearing area for maxillary denture

Ans. Rugae area

392. What is relief area in all the cases?

Ans. Maxillary tuberosity

393. Name a non-limiting area?

Ans. Maxillary tuberosity

397. Give an example of oro-facial region that is not considered a relief area?

Ans. Palatine fovea region

395. The support for maxillary denture is provided mainly by

Ans. Hard palate

396. Name the muscle that is not associated with maxillary buccal frenum

Ans. Masseter

397. Which muscle pulls maxillary buccal frenum forward during function of mandible?

Ans. Orbicularis oris

398. Which muscle pulls maxillary frenum backward during functional activities of mandible?

Ans. Buccinator

399. Buccal vestibule distally extends up to

Ans. Hamular notch

400. Posterior vibrating line is

Ans. Always on soft palate

401. The upper denture must extend distally

Ans. Either to the posterior vibrating line or 1–2 mm posterior to it

402. The connective tissue layer of mucous membrane is known as

Ans. Lamina propria

403. Which is the primary stress bearing area for the maxillary complete denture?

Ans. Horizontal portion of the hard palate lateral to midline

404. As the resorption takes place, the incisive foramen

Ans. Lies close to crest of the residual ridge

405. What is role of enlarged maxillary tuberosity?

Ans. It prevents proper location of the occlusal plane and it may interfere with the lower denture

406. Torus palatinus is found in about

Ans. 20% of the population

407. Which muscle is present beneath the buccal frenum?

Ans. Levator anguli oris

408. The root of the zygoma is located

Ans. Opposite to maxillary 1st molar

409. Vibrating line is about

Ans. 2 mm in front of fovea palatine

410. What is location of vibrating line?

Ans. It is always present on soft palate

411. The distal end of the maxillary denture should be

Ans. 1–2 mm posterior to vibrating line

412. Given an example of relief area?

Ans. Midpalatal sutural area

413. The material of choice for preliminary impression is

Ans. Alginate

414. How much larger should be the metal stock tray than the outer surface of residual ridge for alginate impression material?

Ans. Approximately 5 mm

415. The dimensions of posterior palatal seal are

Ans. 1–1.5 mm high x 1.5 mm broad

416. The thickness of the custom tray should be

Ans. 2–3 mm

417. Which area on the cast is not covered by spacer during construction of custom tray?

Ans. Posterior palatal seal area

418. For the purpose of border molding, the flanges of custom tray should be

Ans. 2 mm short of the tissue reflections

419. The border reduction from inner, outer and top surfaces of border molded custom tray for final impression material is

Ans. 0.5 mm approximately

420. Limiting structure of mandibular denture is

Ans. Retromolar fossa and pad

421. Distally and laterally the buccal shelf is bounded by

Ans. Retromolar pad and external oblique ridge respectively

422. The direction of vertical occlusal forces to the buccal shelf area is

Ans. Vertical

423. The primary stress-bearing area for lower denture is

Ans. Buccal shelf area

424. The buccinators muscle fibers run in the buccal shelf just overlying the bone

Ans. Horizontally in anteroposterior direction

425. Distobuccal corner of lower denture is made to converge rapidly to allow

Ans. Contraction of masseter muscle

426. If distobuccal corner of lower denture is not made to converge than denture is displaced by

Ans. Masseter muscle

427. Anteriorly the mylohyoid muscle lies

Ans. Deep to sublingual glands

428. Which of the region, is not influenced by the mylohyoid muscle?

Ans. Retromylohyoid fossa

429. Which muscle causes bulge in the wall of retromylohyoid curtain?

Ans. Medial pterygoid

430. The middle part of lingual flange of lower denture curves

Ans. Medially

431. Lingual flange of denture is made to extend below the level of mylohyoid ridge in

Ans. Middle region of alveololingual sulcus

432. Space exists between inner surface of lingual flange and mylohyoid muscle when

Ans. Mylohyoid muscle is contracted and tongue is protruded

433. The mylohyoid muscle attachment extends distally

Ans. Up to about one cm back of mylohyoid ridge

434. In case of extremely resorbed lower ridge, the numbness of lower lip is most probably due to

Ans. Compression of metal nerves and vessels

435. If the final impressions are made in tray with no space for impression material, the technique is termed as

Ans. Pressure impression technique

436. Which area is not covered by spacer in lower custom tray?

Ans. Buccal shelf and retromylohyoid fossa

437. Name one temporary recording base material?

Ans. Vinyl or polystyrene

438. What needs refractory cast for fabrication of recording bases?

Ans. Cast alloys

439. The occlusal plane of occlusion rims should be parallel to

Ans. Chamfer line and interpupillary line

440. Corners of the mouth provide anterior stable landmarks for the height of

Ans. Mandibular first premolar

441. Which tooth has its level of occlusal plane is at the junction of inferior two third and superior one third of retromolar pad?

Ans. Mandibular first molar

442. The silverman's space for most class-I patients is about

Ans. 1.5–3 mm

443. The ideal height of anterior maxillary occlusion rim from the reflection of the cast should be approximately

Ans. 22 mm

444. The ideal height of anterior mandibular occlusion rim from the reflection of the cast should be approximately

Ans. 16 mm

445. The level of maxillary occlusal rim in the first molar area should be below the Stensen duct by approximately

Ans. 6 mm

446. What can locate the axis of mandibular rotation in sagittal plane?

Ans. Orientation jaw relation

447. What is related to cranium?

Ans. Orientation jaw relation

448. What is related to jaw separation?

Ans. Vertical relation

449. In retruded position of mandible, the heads of the condyles can only

Ans. Rotate

450. Rotation of condyles takes place in

Ans. Lower compartment of temporomandibular joint

451. Face-bow is used to record the

Ans. Opening axis (Hinge axis)

452. Which is most commonly used in complete denture construction?

Ans. Arbitrary face-bow

453. The condyle rods of arbitrary face-bow are placed on cantho-tragal line in front of external auditory meatus at a distance of

Ans. About 13 mm from external auditory meatus

454. At what distance from the true opening axis of the condyle rods of arbitrary face-bow are placed?

Ans. Within 5 mm

455. Whose fork is attached to maxillary occlusal rim

Ans. Arbitrary face-bow

456. Condyle rods of which type of face-bow are located on true centre of opening axis of the jaws?

Ans. Kinematic face-bow

457. Whose condyle rods donot fit into the external auditory meatus

Ans. Hanau face-bow

458. What determines the arbitrary axis within 2 mm of true centre of opening axis of mandible?

Ans. Hanau face-bow

459. The face-bow scale of Denar slidematic face-bow represents

Ans. Half the patient's intercondylar distance

460. Multiple transfer jigs may be used with only one

Ans. Slidematic face-bow

461. What remains relatively constant for reasonable length of time?

Ans. Physiologic rest position of mandible

462. Interocclusal distance in physiologic rest position of mandible in premolar area of class-I patient is normally

Ans. 2–4 mm

463. In cases of narrow knife-edge ridges, complete dentures become more comfortable if made with

Ans. Increased interocclusal distance

464. If the interarch distance is reduced than

Ans. Corners of the mouth turn down

465. Clicking of complete dentures is most probably due to

Ans. Increased vertical height and failure to provide inter occlusal distance

466. In natural dentition the incisal edges of mandibular anterior teeth are vertically apart from the incisive papilla by approximately

Ans. 4 mm

467. Orientation relation establishes the references in

Ans. Cranium

468. Face-bow is used for

Ans. Recording of orientation relation

469. Arbitrary face bow is mostly used

Ans. For complete denture

470. Decrease in vertical dimension of the occlusion results in

Ans. Decreased muscle tone

471. Which is not a mechanical method for determining the vertical maxillomandibular relations?

Ans. Phonetics and esthetics

472. The incisal edges of the maxillary anterior teeth from incisive papilla are approximately

Ans. 6 mm

473. On an average the interocclusal gap at rest position in premolar area is

Ans. 2–4 mm

474. Jaw relationships are classified into

Ans. Three groups

475. Occlusion rims are attached to which part of the face bow?

Ans. Fork

476. Which face bow is usually used in edentulous patients?

Ans. Arbitrary face-bow

477. The maximum intercuspation of teeth is known as

Ans. Centric occlusion

478. Centric occlusion is

Ans. 1 mm anterior to centric relation

479. The development of distal spaces between the upper and lower occlusal surfaces of the occlusion rims or denture in protrusion is known as

Ans. Christensen phenomenon

480. Lateral condylar path inclination is approximately

Ans. 15°

481. The coble device can be used for recording

Ans. Horizontal jaw relations only

482. Name an intraoral tracing device?

Ans. Coble device

483. Gliding movements of the mandible take place in

Ans. Upper compartment of the temporomandibular joint

484. Jaw movements are studied by

Ans. Pantograph

485. The interocclusal distance is also known as

Ans. Freeway space

486. The interocclusal gap in class I cases is

Ans. 2–4 mm

487. The interocclusal gap in class II cases is

Ans. More than 4 mm

488. Condylar guidance in arcon articulator is located in

Ans. Upper member on the articular

489. Hanau model 130-28 articulator is

Ans. Semi adjustable articulator

490. The lateral movement of the mandible is known as

Ans. Bennett shift

491. The Bennett shift is approximately

Ans. 15°

492. In the selection of the artifical teeth, what needs to be selected first?

Ans. Color of the tooth

493. Which teeth should be used in the patient with highly visible gingiva?

Ans. Square teeth with long contact point

494. Which type of tooth should be used in dentures opposing natural dentition?

Ans. Acrylic

495. The buccolingual width of posterior artificial teeth as compared to natural teeth should be?

Ans. Less than natural teeth

496. Which type of teeth are used when they oppose the natural teeth whose occlusal surfaces are restored with gold?

Ans. Acrylic teeth and composite teeth

497. Which teeth are desirable when the tooth must be excessively reduced in height because of small interarch distance?

Ans. Acrylic teeth

498. Which teeth are chemically bonded to the acrylic denture bases?

Ans. Acrylic teeth

499. When the residual ridge undergoes resorption, the crest of the ridge

Ans. Is posterior as compared in patient with recent extraction

500. When the teeth are set over the ridge with excessive residual ridge resorption, it will result in

Ans. Prematurely aged appearance

501. The incisal edge of the maxillary central incisor should be

Ans. 0.5 mm below the wax occlusal rim level

502. The proper arrangement of the maxillary and mandibular anterior and posterior teeth depends on the setting of

Ans. Maxillary central incisor

503. The incisal tip of the mandibular canine should be

Ans. At the occlusal rim level

504. The artificial anterior teeth should be essentially placed

Ans. At the same position previously occupied natural teeth

505. If the occlusal plane is too low anteriorly or too high posteriorly, the maxillary denture will

Ans. Slide anteriorly

506. The 'neutral zone' concept was given by

Ans. Fish

507. What causes anterior displacement of denture?

Ans. The setting of posterior teeth on residual ridge incline as it ascends towards retromolar pad

508. If due to the availability of less space in mandibular posterior region only three teeth are to be used, which posterior tooth should be dropped?

Ans. Mandibular 1st premolar

509. Which mandibular tooth should be according to setting of maxillary teeth?

Ans. Mandibular 1st premolar

510. The mediolateral compensating curve is how many degrees from the horizontal plane of orientation?

Ans. 5°–10°

511. A high condylar guidance requires

Ans. Greater compensating curve

512. The working side interferences will be found on

Ans. Lingual inclines of facial cusps

513. Examples of supporting cusps one

Ans. Maxillary lingual and mandibular lingual cusps

514. The supporting cusps of maxillary posterior teeth articulate with

Ans. Central fossae of mandibular posterior teeth and marginal ridges of mandibular posterior teeth

515. Before the jaw relation records are perfected and verified at the time of try in appointment, the patient should be advised to leave the old denture out of the mouth for a minimum period of

Ans. 24 hours

516. The incisal guidance is determined by

Ans. Both horizontal and vertical overlap of anterior teeth

517. The minimum amount of protrusion for condylar guidance advancement is

Ans. 6 mm

518. Foveae palatine are

Ans. Coalescence of ducts

519. The vibrating line may be located

Ans. Slightly anterior to the foveae palatine

520. The width of the posterior palatal seal is usually

Ans. 1–1.5 mm

521. When the posterior palatal seal is made too wide (usual width is 1–1.5 mm) it will result in

Ans. Downward displacement of the denture

522. The vertical groove in the middle of upper lip is called as

Ans. Philtrum

523. Which muscle does not merge with orbicularis oris muscle?

Ans. Masseter

524. Which factor affects the repositioning of the orbicularis oris muscle with complete dentures?

Ans. The amount of separation between mandible and maxille

525. In which dental arch forms the central incisors are at greater distance forward from the canines?

Ans. Tapering arch

526. High 'V' shaped edentulous vault indicates

Ans. Tapering dental arch

527. Buccal corridor is the space between

Ans. Buccal surface of upper teeth and corner of the mouth

528. The vertical position of which tooth is responsible for the shape of the smiling line?

Ans. Maxillary canine

529. The dentogenic concept of facial and functional harmony was considered by

Ans. Frush and Fisher

530. Which anterior tooth is more distally inclined at cervical end than other teeth?

Ans. Maxillary lateral incisor

531. Which tooth is more prominent at the cervical end?

Ans. Maxillary canine

532. Which material is most commonly used in the fabrication of the complete denture?

Ans. Heat curing acrylic resins

533. How much thickness of denture base is desirable over retromolar pad and maxillary tuberosity to avoid interference?

Ans. 1.5 mm

534. Which material should be ideally used for flasking?

Ans. Dental stone

535. Dewaxing in boiling water should be done for maximum of

Ans. 3–5 minutes

536. How much powder liquid ratio is used in acrylic resin denture fabrication?

Ans. 3 1

537. The excess amount of resin dough, which comes out of flask during packing, is called as?

Ans. Flash

538. Before curing cycle begins, ideally the properly packed flask should be allowed to stand for

Ans. 30–60 minutes

539. The specified curing cycle temperature and time is

Ans. 165°F and 9 hours and 165°F for 90 minutes followed by 30 minutes at boil

540. Fluid resin is a type of

Ans. Chemically polymerized acrylic resin

541. Which material does not contain methyl methacrylate?

Ans. Visible light activated composites

542. What is a disadvantage of metal denture base?

Ans. Greater weight

543. Centric relation is a

Ans. Bone to bone relation

544. Centric occlusion is a

Ans. Tooth to tooth relation

545. The errors in occlusion should be eliminated

Ans. On the articulator

546. The selective grinding done in the mouth according to articulating paper marks usually results in

Ans. Decreased amount of error in the occlusion

547. After centric occlusion has been perfected, which cusps should not be shortened?

Ans. Lingual cusps of maxillary and buccal cusps of mandibular teeth

548. When carborundum paste is used for correcting errors in centric and eccentric occlusion, it will result in

Ans. Decrease in vertical dimension of occlusion

549. How many types of occlusal errors can occur on working side?

Ans. 6 types

550. What might be responsible for no contact of the teeth on the working side?

Ans. Excessive contact on balancing side

551. Learning to chew satisfactorily with new dentures usually requires at least

Ans. 6–8 weeks

552. What should not be used for the correction of the occlusal errors?

Ans. Carborundum paste

553. The lesion posterior to the hamular notch is usually caused due to

Ans. Long denture borders

554. The excessive pressure from the mandibular buccal flange in the region of the mental foramen may cause tingling sensation in

Ans. Lower lip

555. The excessive pressure on the incisive papilla may cause numbness in

Ans. Anterior part of the hard palate

556. The looseness of maxillary denture on opening mouth wide is caused by

Ans. Thick distobuccal flange of the maxillary denture

557. The clinical procedure which involves adding of small amount of denture material to denture base to compensate the changes that occur in basal seat without adversely affecting the occlusal relationship and esthantics is called as?

Ans. Relining

558. The loss of vertical dimension will cause the mandible to have a

Ans. More forward position in relation to maxilla

559. The pattern of resorption of residual ridge in maxilla is

Ans. Upward and back

560. The pattern of resorption in mandible is

Ans. Downward and forward

561. As the resorption of the residual ridge continues the profile of the face of the patient will become

Ans. Concave

561. By the addition of the tissue conditioner, the strength of the processed resin will

Ans. Decrease

562. The elastic stage of the tissue conditioner is reached in

Ans. 1–2 weeks

563. The lateral condylar guidance can be calculated by

Ans. $L = H/8 + 12$

564. The resistance to removal of a denture in a direction opposite to that of insertion is called as

Ans. Retention

565. The force of attraction between like molecules is called as

Ans. Cohesion

566. Viscous tension was described by

Ans. Stefan

567. Most vulnerable part of alveolar ridge to time-dependent occlusal stresses is

Ans. Posterior mandibular alveolar ridge

568. Which tooth is best overdenture abutment?

Ans. Canine

569. Most common cause of loss of abutment teeth in case of overdenture is

Ans. Periodontal disease

570. Regular follow-up examination of overdenture is needed at intervals of

Ans. 3–6 months

571. How much time is necessary to wear an immediate denture just after extraction?

Ans. 24 hours

572. After how many days of extraction immediate denture can be removed during night?

Ans. Seven days

573. How much bone volume of the ridge is reduced during the first 12 months of extraction?

Ans. 20%–30%

574. How much time is needed by extraction socket to complete its calcification?

Ans. 8–12 months

575. Hard palate is the static roof of

Ans. Oral cavity

576. Surgical resection of posterior part of hard palate generally involves

Ans. Lateral pterygoid muscle

577. Interim obturator prosthesis can serve up to

Ans. Six months

578. Prosthetic goal of interim obturator is

Ans. Restore deglutition and restore speech

579. Surgical obturator prosthesis will be in service for approximately

Ans. Five days